HOW
TO
BE
PLUMP

HOW
TO
BE
PLUMP

·

A Victorian Re-creation

·

by
Reinier Beeuwkes III
and Rhonda Poe

E. P. DUTTON NEW YORK

This book is an abridged and illustrated version of *How to Be Plump: Or Talks on Physiological Feeding,* by T. C. Duncan, M.D., published by Duncan Brothers, Chicago, in 1878.

The text was prepared by Reinier Beeuwkes III. The book was designed and illustrated by Rhonda Poe, using engravings from period sources as republished in the Dover Pictorial Archives Series. Typography by Berkeley Associates of Bala Cynwyd, Pennsylvania.

Published in the United States by E. P. Dutton,
a division of NAL Penguin Inc.,
2 Park Avenue, New York, N.Y. 10016.

Published simultaneously in Canada by Fitzhenry and Whiteside,
Limited, Toronto.

Library of Congress Catalog Card Number: 88-70163

ISBN: 0-525-24683-5

10 9 8 7 6 5 4 3 2 1

First Edition

"...you'll find that as you get wider, you'll get wiser. Width and wisdom, Sammy, always grows together."

Charles Dickens
Pickwick Papers

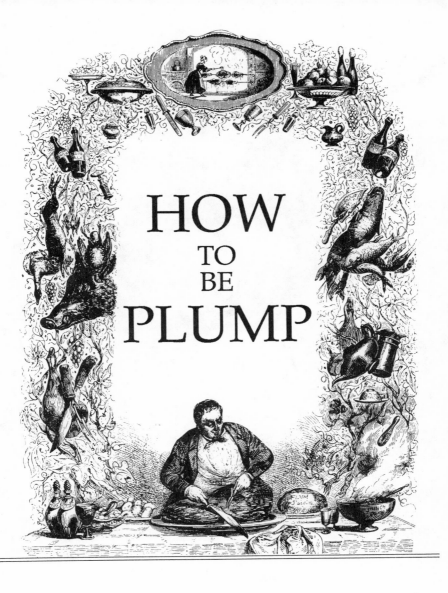

HOW
TO
BE
PLUMP

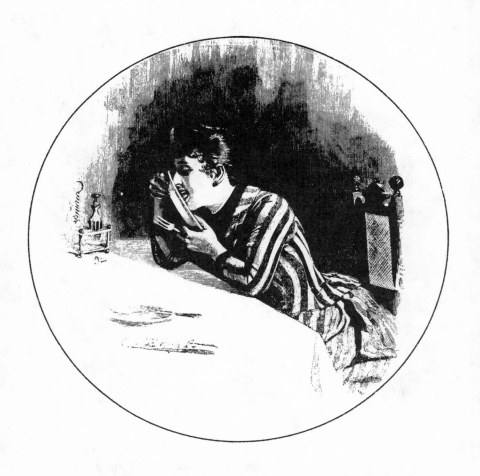

TABLE OF CONTENTS

PAGE

Preface... 3

Introduction.. 4

CHAPTER I.
How I Became Plump.................................... 6

CHAPTER II.
Leanness a Disease.. 14

CHAPTER III.
The Importance of Fat.................................. 26

CHAPTER IV.
The Importance of Starchy Food and Sweets........... 32

CHAPTER V.
How to Become Plump.................................. 39

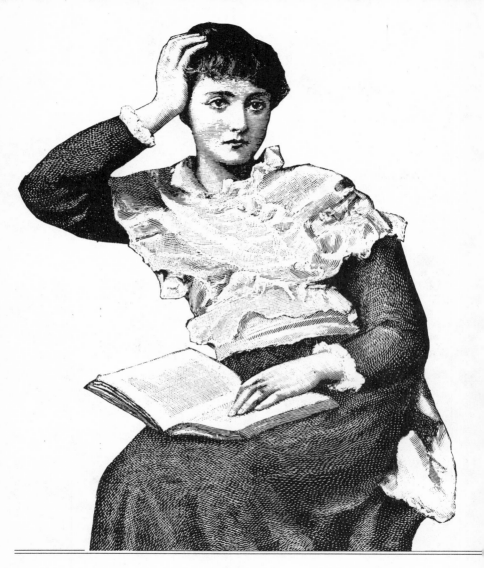

PREFACE

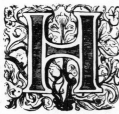ow shall I get fleshy? "I would give a dollar a pound for more fat!" "This climate agrees with me nicely; I never was so well and fleshy in my life." "I have fleshed up remarkably this year and feel, oh, so much better!" "Weighed one hundred and forty pounds, I felt well; now I weigh only one hundred and ten pounds, and feel so miserable!"

Why is plumpness associated with health, and leanness with disease? Why are "Americans proverbially lean?" These are vital questions that touch the philanthropic, interest the statesman, and arouse scientific investigations. The following pages have been prepared with the hope that they may prove as valuable to every lean person as their personal application has been to

THE AUTHOR

INTRODUCTION

uring the last ten years, the question of feeding has been one to which I have given much thought. The quieting effect of a few pounds of fat gave me a clue to much of the restless activity of Americans. The fact that thin children are imperfectly developed as adults was an observation that lifted a dark cloud of suspicion from the holy

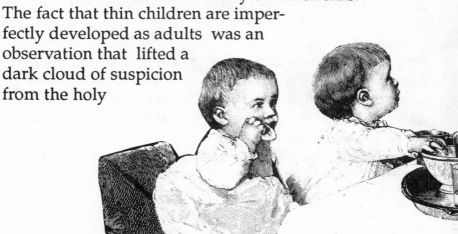

atmosphere of American motherhood. It was a happy relief when I found that fat would delay and perfect development.

If the perusal of these pages will enable a mother to keep her children fat, fair and rosy; to assist any young lady to keep plump and well; to prevent any rushing business man from breaking down for the want of a good bank account of fat laid up for emergencies; or in any way con- duce to the happiness of man- kind, this little work will have fulfilled an important mission.

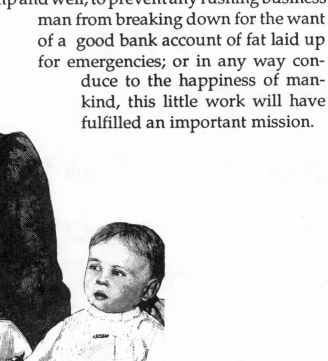

CHAPTER I.

How I Became Plump.

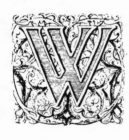ell, doctor, I declare, how fleshy you are getting, I guess you practice the maxim: Laugh and grow fat!"

"No, I laugh because I am fleshy and feel buoyant."

"Well, tell me how you became fleshy?"

"It is not a long story. Some winters ago I had a patient in the oyster trade. He came to see me almost every day, and always brought a can or two of oysters."

"I did not know that oysters were fattening. How did you cook them?"

"Well, in almost every shape, but generally in a stew."

"Why did not Mrs. Duncan get fleshy also?"

"Well, she never eats hearty, does not like oyster stews, and always puts vinegar and pepper on her oysters."

"Do vinegar and pepper interfere with getting fat?"

"Acids quicken the circulation, and unduly excite the system."

"So excitement prevents fattening?"

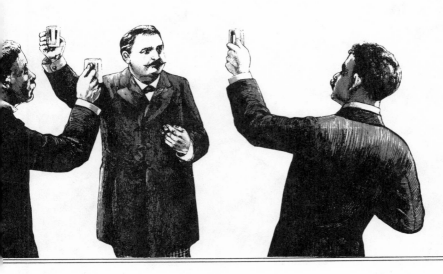

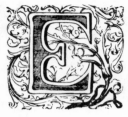xcitement takes away the appetite by unduly stimulating the brain. I have seen nervous women go weeks without eating enough to keep a bird alive."

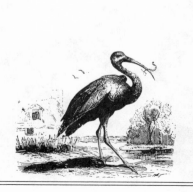

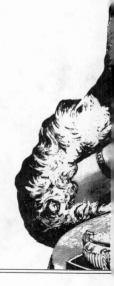

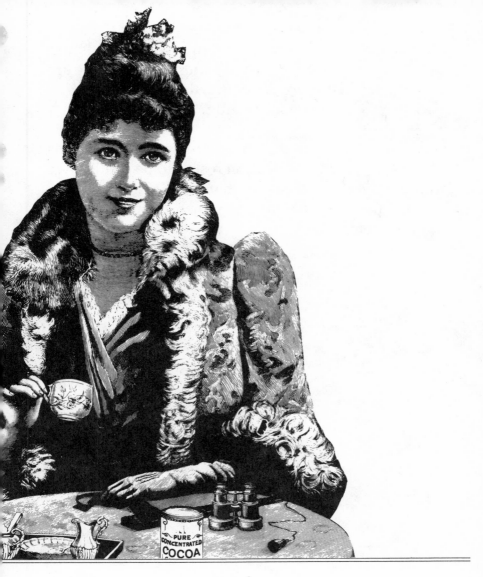

ou say that stimulants, spices, acids and activity prevent fattening. As there are rules for fattening, then must there be a science in feeding?"

"There is a scientific basis on which this whole question rests. To be healthy we want to know what to eat, so that we may observe the golden mean - *florid plumpness*, which is the picture of health the world over."

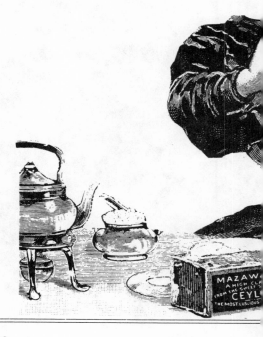

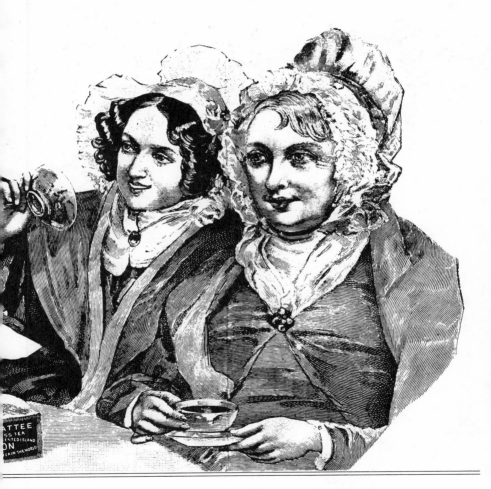

n your own case you found these rules. Now will you tell me how to get plump?"

"I will be very glad indeed to accommodate you. I have told you what to avoid, now I will tell you what to eat. Water, starchy food, fats, vegetables, sweets, and quiet: these put on the fat."

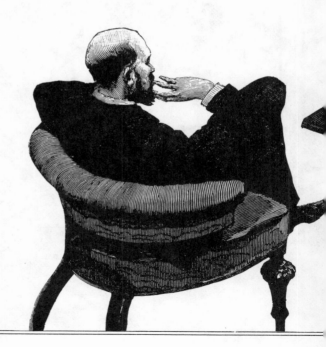

"That is it! Just as we did to fatten pigs when I was a boy. Shut them in a small pen and gave them all they would eat of corn and slops."

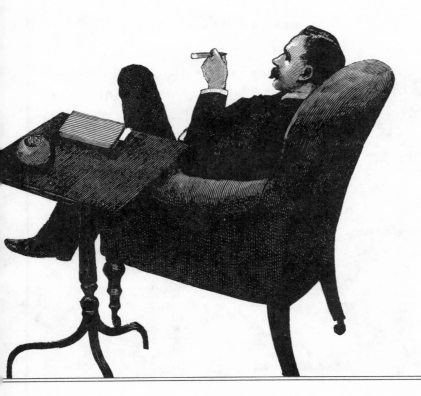

CHAPTER II.

Leanness a Disease.

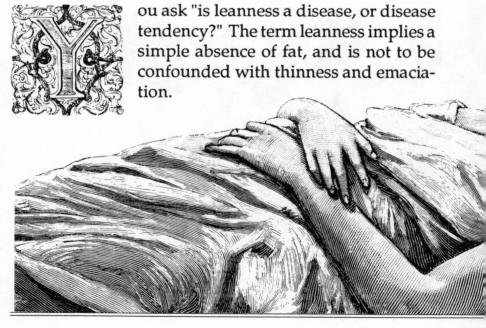

ou ask "is leanness a disease, or disease tendency?" The term leanness implies a simple absence of fat, and is not to be confounded with thinness and emaciation.

Leanness, when it cannot be referred to a satisfactory cause, must be accounted a disease. When extreme, it must almost always be considered as morbid.

Almost any change for the worse in health is at once betrayed in most people by a loss of fat. On the other hand, the gain of fat up to a certain point seems to go hand in hand with a rise in all other essentials of health.

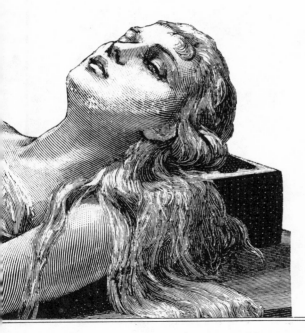

he causes of leanness may be climate or locality; and diet and exercise. The inhabitants of mountainous and barren sandy regions are naturally disposed to be lean.

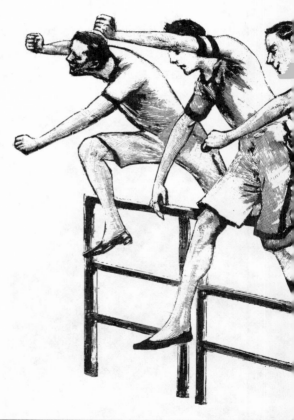

Leanness, more than from any other cause, results from a deficient diet and *excessive bodily exercise.*

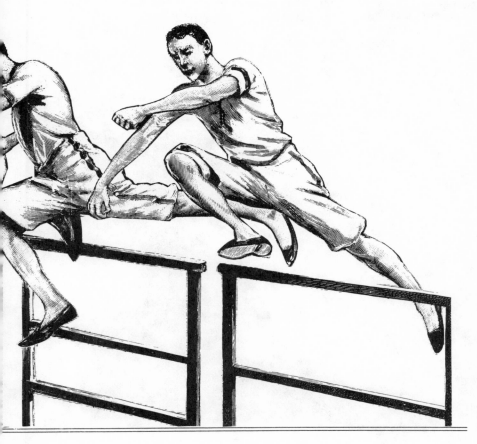

n spare individuals fat is disposed of as fast as it is deposited, so as to prevent its accumulation. This particularly occurs in healthy individuals who are mentally worried, and who under no system of diet whatever, would become fat.

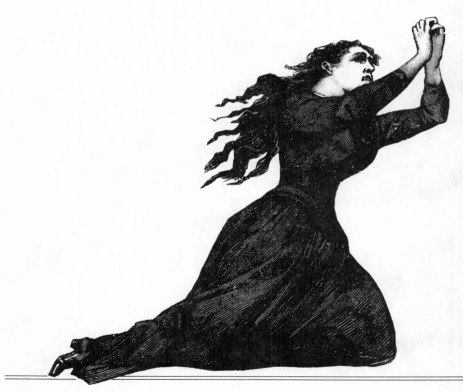

There is a restless anxiety about lean people that is distressing. They look hungry, sad and irritable.

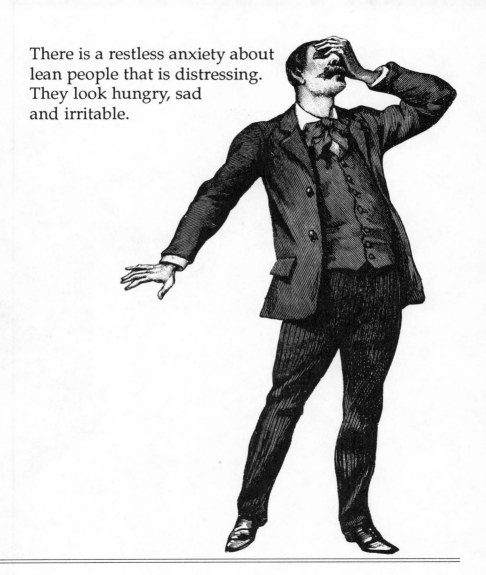

n the lean, the functions are performed with difficulty, friction is manifest everywhere, and there are often explosions of the nervous system.

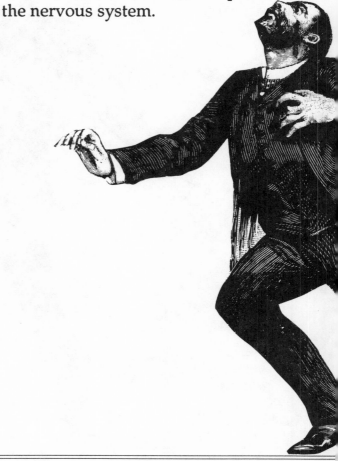

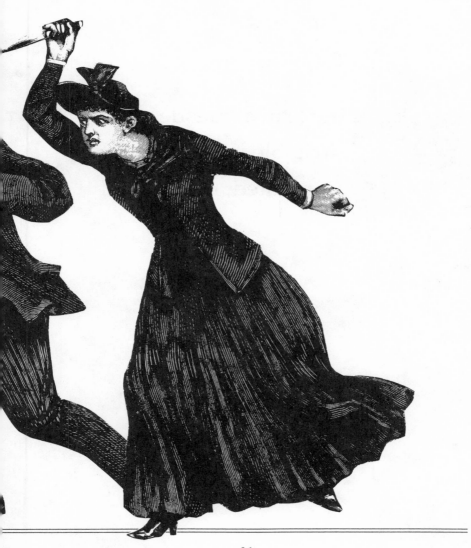

he lean are restless and irritable in mind, rarely contented, never quiet . . .

They form the complaining element of society, and are unstable as a nation.

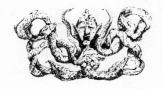

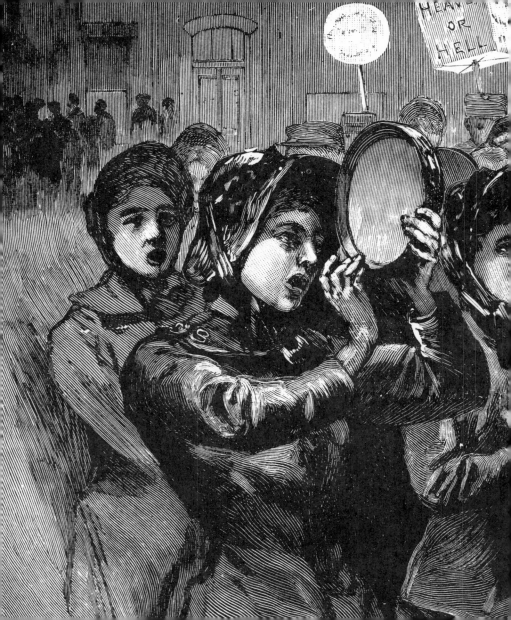

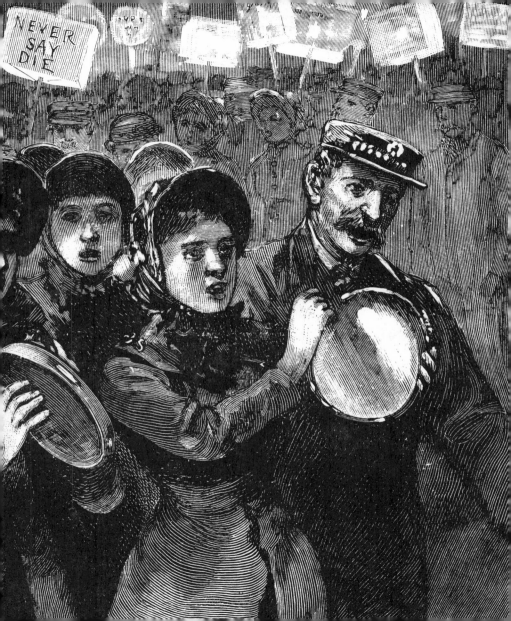

CHAPTER III.

The Importance of Fat.

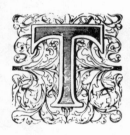he importance of fat is physical, mental and moral. A child well nourished, fat and fair, grows rapidly and develops easily. A child thin in flesh develops poorly and with a struggle.

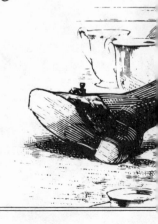

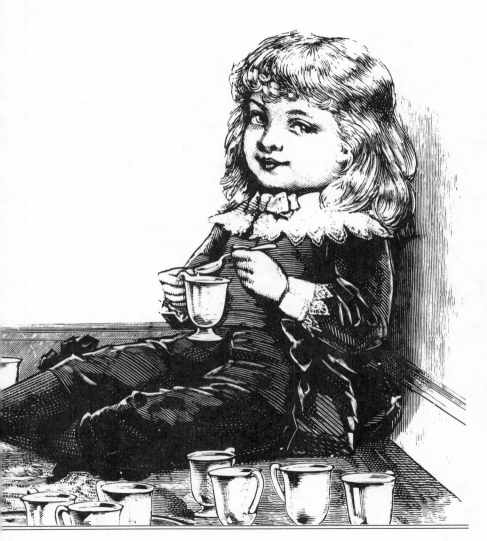

he instinctive desire shown by all nations for an oily diet, and the association of this substance with the ideas of luxury in all times, shows the value of fat to man's comfort. The "butter and honey" of the prophet, used as a phrase for royal food, and the reference in almost every other page of the Bible to oil as a luxury, are sufficient to show its estimation.

In the lean the organs are poorly nourished, there is no fat in the abdomen, and the form bends and contracts as in old age, while the fleshy body stands nobly erect and has a royal mien.

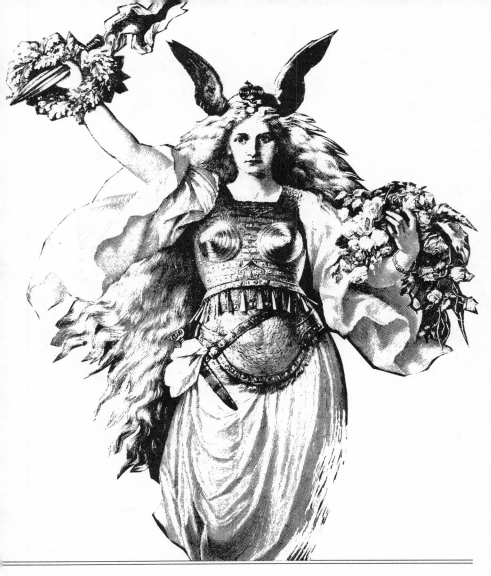

he great importance of sufficient fat is not properly appreciated. Fat is found in nearly all parts of the body; it aids digestion and assimilation, quickens the circulation, and hastens cell activity. That fat admits of high organization is evident from the large proportion in the cerebral and nervous tissues. One-fourth at least of the solid matter composing the brain is said to consist of fats.

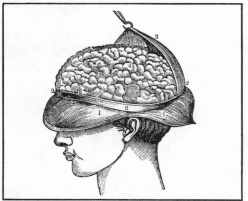

Fat, as a nonconducting substance, is very necessary in cold weather in impeding escape of animal heat.

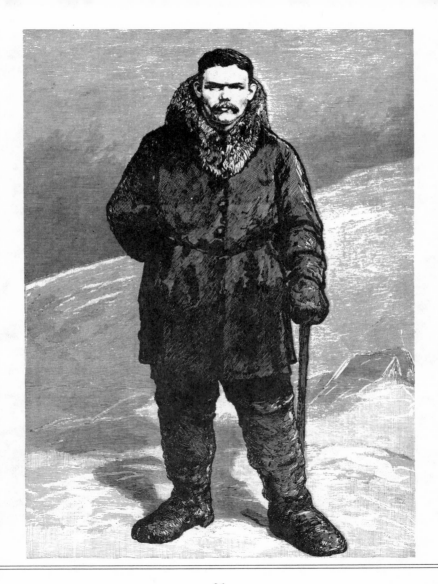

CHAPTER IV.

The Importance of Starchy Food and Sweets.

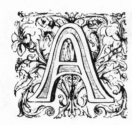 re starchy food and sweets fattening?"

It is well known that sweets aid in the fattening process. In sugar

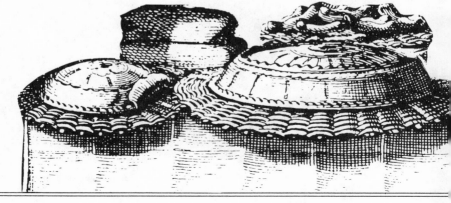

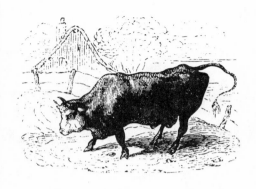

growing countries the cattle employed on the planta-
tions grow remarkably stout, while the cane is being
gathered and the sugar extracted. During this harvest
the saccharine juices are freely consumed; but when the
season is over the superabundant adipose tissue is
gradually lost.

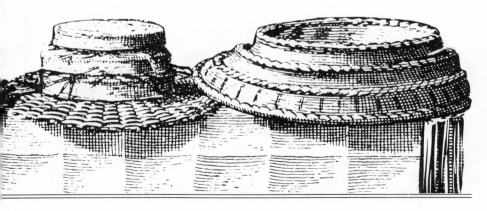

n the Orient the women of the harem are fattened, against a certain day...

by feeding them freely with
honey and black bread.

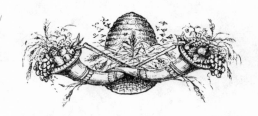

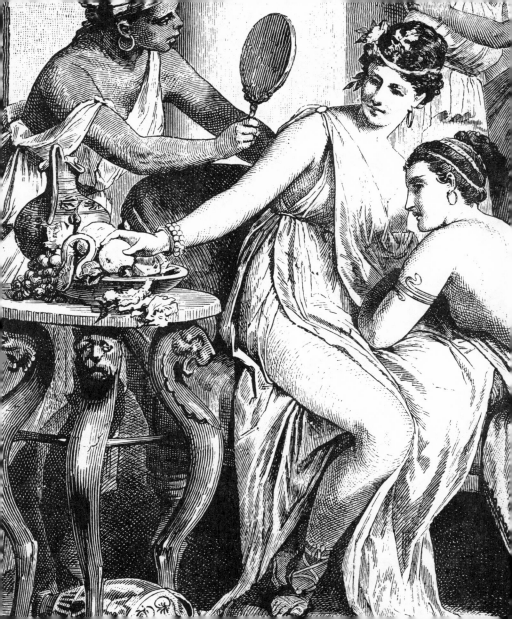

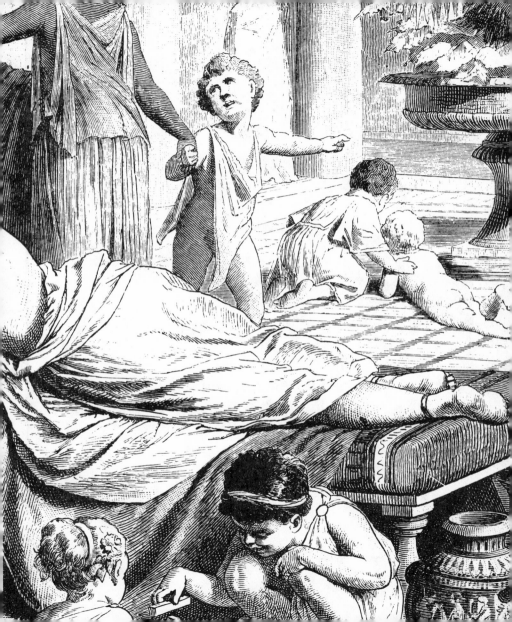

CHAPTER V.

How to Become Plump.

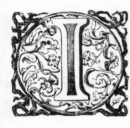n the first chapter I told you how I became plump. I began to eat oysters as a steady diet, day after day. I noticed that after taking oyster stews with supper, I began to bloat about the waist. This bloating was rather distressing at first, and I became a little concerned. I have often had the same uncomfortable, distended feeling after a hearty meal of substantial food, but no serious result followed.

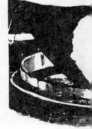

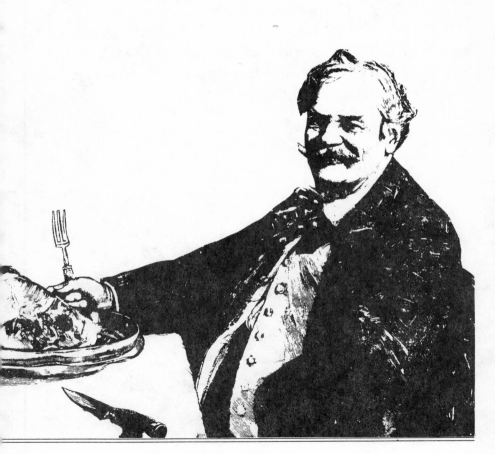

I soon learned that bloating was the first step in the fattening process. We must "bloat up," then "fat up." This bloating is often very uncomfortable, and some ladies have suddenly abandoned their plans laid down for fattening, on its appearance. But a little perseverance in the fattening diet soon changes all this for plump bodies, rounded limbs and full faces.

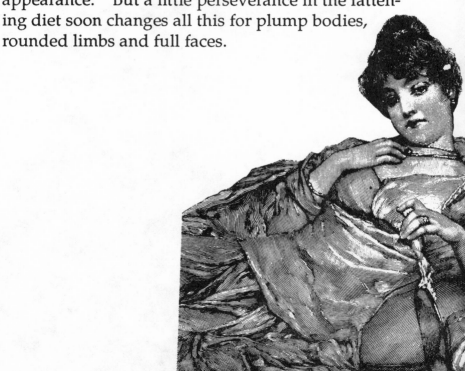

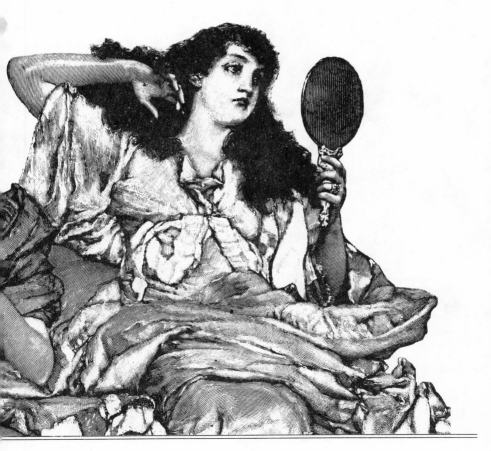

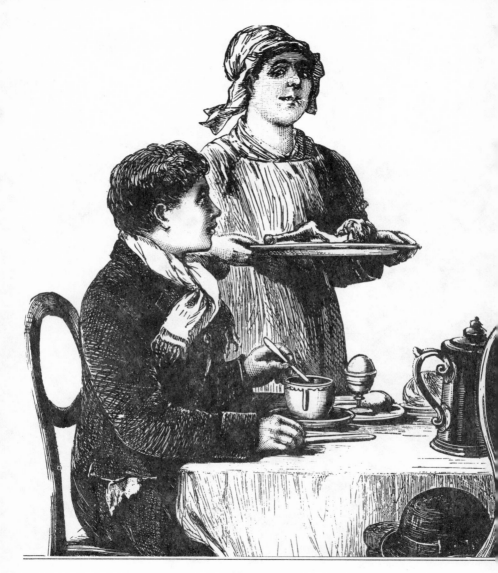

he breakfast should be plain and substantial, and should be hearty the year round, especially in summer. "Egg on toast, with a cup of coffee" is not enough. Potatoes, meat, (fried mush or oat meal porridge, is a good substitute), bread and butter, with some form of drink should be taken. There is no serious objection to tea or coffee if they are well "milked."

he hearty meal of the day should come four hours - not later than five hours - after breakfast. The first thing taken should be a light soup, not highly seasoned. Soup reinforces the digestive juices. Vegetables should enter largely into this meal. Condiments, spices, acids and stimulants, unless very mild, should be avoided. Cold water should also be eschewed, as it chills the stomach and thoroughly weakens it. The drink should be chocolate or milk.

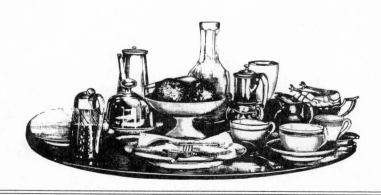

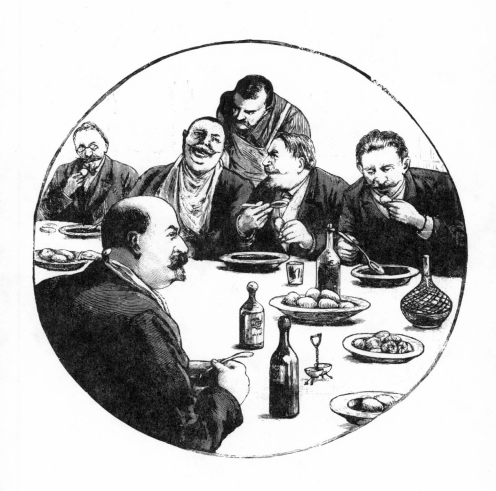

 he evening meal should be light. Bread and milk, or oat meal mush and milk is almost too substantial. A hearty meal at this hour clogs the circulation, and makes sleep heavy and unrefreshing. This meal should be eaten slowly with pleasant company.

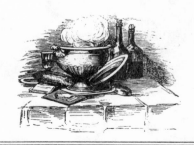

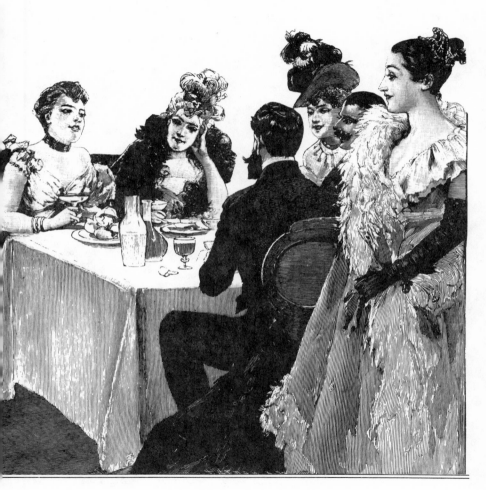

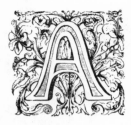ctivity of mind or body prevents fat-
tening. Sufficient rest must be
secured.

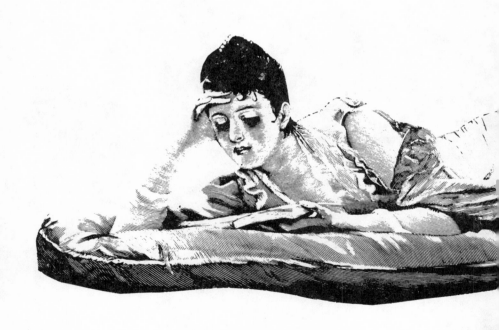

Persons who want to get and keep plump, must give the system time to recruit. They should retire about 10 P.M. and enjoy sleep until 6 or 7 A.M. Children and old people should retire early.

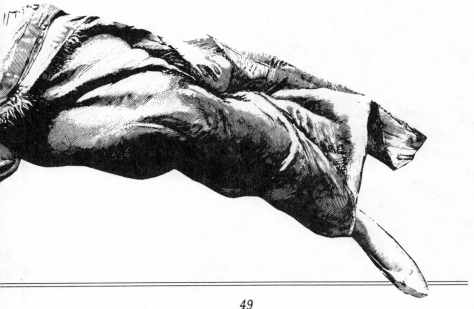

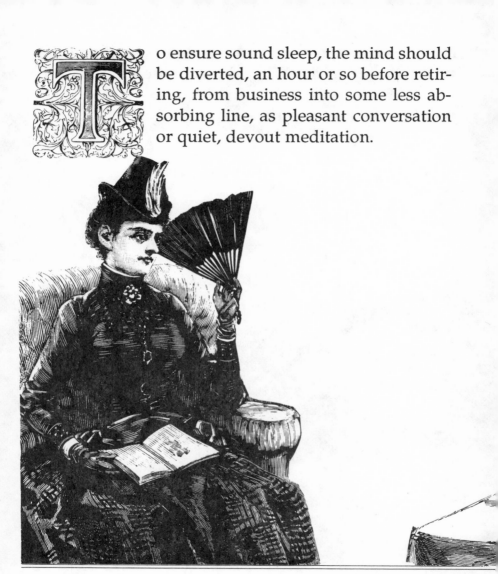

o ensure sound sleep, the mind should be diverted, an hour or so before retiring, from business into some less absorbing line, as pleasant conversation or quiet, devout meditation.

Those who cannot divert the mind will be apt to break down, and will be very hard to fatten.

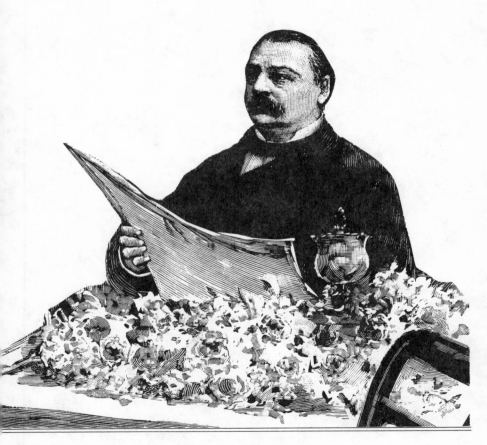

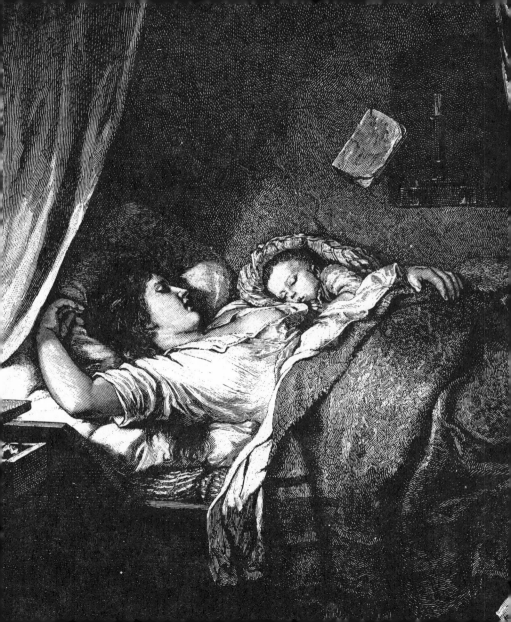

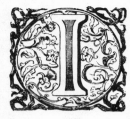f a habit of night-work has been acquired, it should be broken up as speedily as possible. The fact that consumptives, as a rule, are "owls," should be evidence enough that night-work of any kind is too consuming. There is more truth than poetry in the maxim,

"Early to bed and early to rise
Make a man *healthy*, wealthy and wise."

FINIS

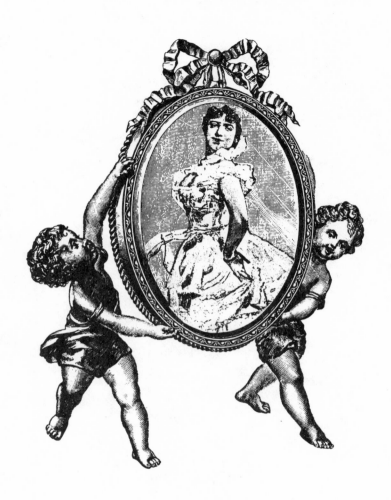